Permanently Beat Yeast Infection & Candida

Proven Step-by-Step Cure for Yeast Infections & Candidiasis, Natural, Lasting Treatment That Will Prevent Recurring Infection [Plus FREE Bonus eBook!]

Caroline D. Greene

Published by Women's Republic

Atlanta, Georgia USA

WOMEN'S
Republic

ISBN 978-1-48396-787-5

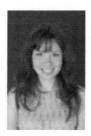

Copyright © 2012 Caroline D. Greene

What Our Readers Are Saying

"In just a few hours, my single most unpleasant symptom had gone - fantastic!"

★★★★★Emily S. (Lakeview, OR)

"I'm just so relieved to know that there is an effective treatment and that there is an end in sight!"

★★★★★Rachel V. (Newry, SC)

"I almost felt cheated when I saw how simple and natural the cure was...but then it worked! Thank you, thank you, thank you!"

★★★★★Keisha P. (Hoffman, MN)

"It was a nice change to get a product that did exactly what it claimed it would"

★★★★☆Judith R. (Johnstown, PA)

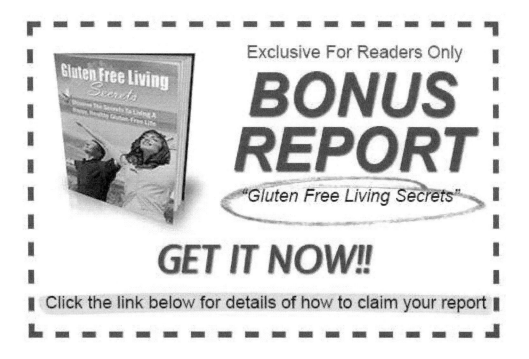

Exclusive Bonus Download: Gluten Free Living Secrets

Are you sick and tired of trying every weight loss program out there and failing to see results? Or are you frustrated with not feeling as energetic as you used to despite what you eat? Perhaps you always seem to have a bit of a " dodgy stomach " and indigestion seems to be a regular part of your life?

There's nothing worse than sitting down to a nice big plate of pasta and enjoying your meal only to be met with a growling stomach and the inevitable rush to the toilet.

It's that bloated feeling you get after eating a piece of bread that just " doesn't seem right " . Almost as if you've eaten something poisonous.

Gluten Free Living Secrets is a complete resource that will tell you everything you need to know about the dangers of eating gluten and how to go about transitioning yourself and your family to a life free of this dangerous substance.

Here's just a taste of what you will discover inside Gluten Free Living Secrets:

- What foods you should focus on when first switching to a gluten-free diet
- The 9 grains that are safe and gluten-free
- The truth about whether you can eat pasta on a gluten-free diet

- What you should know to determine if you have Celiac Disease

- and that's not all...

- Why you may want to consider eliminating gluten from your child's diet

- The top 10 reasons to go gluten-free

- How to transform your pantry to be gluten-free

- A list of essential gluten-free shopping tips

- How to keep your kids happy around their gluten-eating friends

- Tips on staying gluten-free when eating out

Go to the end of this book for the download link for this Bonus!

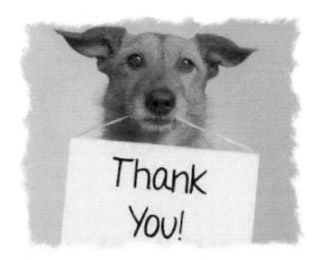

Thank you for downloading my book. Please REVIEW this book on Amazon. I need your feedback to make the next version better. Thank you so much!

Books by This Author

Permanently Beat Bacterial Vaginosis

Permanently Beat Yeast Infection & Candida

Permanently Beat Urinary Tract Infections

Permanently Beat Hypothyroidism Naturally

Permanently Beat PCOS

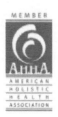

TABLE OF CONTENTS

Disclaimer

While all attempts have been made to provide effective, verifiable information in this Book, neither the Author nor Publisher assumes any responsibility for errors, inaccuracies, or omissions. Any slights of people or organizations are unintentional.

This Book is not a source of medical information, and it should not be regarded as such. This publication is designed to provide accurate and authoritative information in regard to the subject matter covered. It is sold with the understanding that the publisher is not engaged in rendering a medical service. As with any medical advice, the reader is strongly encouraged to seek professional medical advice before taking action.

Chapter 1: Understanding Yeast Infections

What Is A Yeast Infection?

Yeast infections or candidiasis (pronounced: can-dih-die-uh-sis) are surprisingly common and more than 75% of women will experience at least one episode at some point in their lives with almost half of women having two or more vaginal yeast infections within their lifetime.

These infections are caused by a fungus known as Candida albicans which is a member of the yeast family. This is found in small amounts within the digestive tract, the skin, the mouth and also inside the vagina. It is known as one of the pathogenic species of yeasts which, very unlike the friendly species which are known by the name probiotics, can impact negatively upon one's health and can also cause infections under certain circumstances. The manifestation of candidias is unpleasant and can at times be painful and uncomfortable too. Usually this condition presents when the immune system is weakened and the bacterial equilibrium is upset.

Where it can cause problems however is if there is a lack of balance within its living conditions. The fungus then tends to overgrow rapidly within a short space of time and thus begins the yeast infection.

There are various types of yeast infection with the most common being oral candidiasis (commonly known as thrush) and Candidal vulvovaginitis which as the name suggests is vaginal. There are many factors which make a woman more susceptible to this infection, too much sugar and carbohydrate in the diet and long term use of antibiotics can be contributing factors. Candidiasis is also very common and severe in those who have weakened immune systems due to chronic illness.

The most obvious symptom of Oral Thrush is a white, "furry", coated tongue due to the overgrowth of the Candida fungus. Candida can generally be found on the skin and also in mucous membranes. If there is an imbalance within the mouth or throat then the Candida may multiply. Generally along with the white tongue sufferers of oral thrush can present with white patches within their throats and mouths. If the fungus is further down within the esophagus, then there may be pain and swallowing difficulties with the potential to cough up little white "bits".

In this book we will concentrate on the vaginal infection as it is the one which most affects women. There can be a stigma with regards to vaginal yeast infections as many people wrongly assume that these are sexually transmitted. Although there is a risk of transferring the yeast infection to a sexual partner if either one of you has candidiasis this is primarily an overgrowth of yeast which begins within an individuals body. If either you or your partner know that you have the infection then it is best to completely refrain from intercourse until it has cleared up. Also you will likely both need to be treated to ensure that you do not pass the yeast infection back and forth.

The reason why we have Candida albicans within our bodies is to seek out and annihilate potentially harmful bacteria. It is there to defend the body against various strains of pathogenic bacteria. Within a normally healthy individual the Candida albicans is controlled by the friendly bacteria within the body and also by the immune system. However, when the immune system is weakened in any way, this results in a significant decrease in the numbers of friendly bacteria and the Candida albicans will then change from yeast to mycelial fungus and will invade the body. The term mycelial is defined as pertaining to the mass of fine branching tubes (hyphae) which form the growth structure of a fungus.

Yeast infections need to be taken care of as soon as one possibly is able to as when it is in its yeast state, Candida is dormant and non-invasive. However in its fungal state it changes completely and becomes invasive and can be difficult to shift without big lifestyle changes.

How Do You Get It?

Candida can overgrow within the body for a plethora of reasons. Anything which affects the immune system such as illness, stress and even pregnancy can be a contributing factor. Medicines such as steroids and also the birth control pill are known to inhibit "good" bacteria within the body thus allowing the yeast to overgrow. Antibiotics, especially tetracyclines are associated with Candida infections and diabetes is also sited as another cause due to the elevated blood sugar of the patient.

Many women who are going through the general hormonal changes and fluctuations at the beginning of their menstrual cycle find that they have a higher tendency to be prone to yeast infections. It is important not to use scented sanitary products at all if you can help it as they are a vaginal irritant. Anything which upsets the healthy bacterial balance of the vagina must also be avoided. Also yeast thrives in a hot and damp environment so ladies should always ensure that they do not wear tight underwear or nylon pantyhose too often to ensure that they keep as healthy as possible and don't give the yeast a chance to multiply.

Many people wrongly associate yeast infections with sexually transmitted diseases and therefore there is somewhat of a stigma with regards to them. Whilst a yeast infection can potentially be passed through sexual intercourse, it is far more likely to come through the other means which have been mentioned previously. It is worth being aware that men can have penile yeast infections too so safe sex is always the best way to minimize your risk of having one transferred to you. The reasons why men get yeast infections are very similar to us ladies, diabetes, diet, antibiotics, a compromised immune system or spermicidal lubricant can potentially be contributory factors.

Here is a quick and non exhaustive list of factors which affect the balance of Candida yeast within the vagina:

- Stress

- Illness

- Menstruation

- Taking the birth control pill

- Taking antibiotics

- Exhaustion

- Lack of sleep

- Eating lots of junk food, particularly sugars

- Taking steroids

- Hormonal changes

- Too tight clothing

- Wearing pantyhose too often

- Using perfumed soaps and deodorants in the vaginal area

- Perfumed toilet paper

- Wearing the same sanitary for long periods without changing it

- Some washing powders can be irritants to individuals

- Using some condoms which have a spermicidal lubricant can adversely affect some sufferers of Candidiasis. Trial and error is recommended and of course the use of regular, non lubricated condoms is to be encouraged!

- Injury

- Pregnancy

- Women who are in wheelchairs can suffer badly from yeast infections as they rarely have enough air circulation as they are most often in a seated position. Speak to your doctor for advice on this is it affects you.

Signs and Symptoms

The symptoms of a yeast infection can differ from person to person and are dependant on whether the overgrowth is mild, moderate or severe. However the early symptoms typically include:

Itching around the genital area - this typically presents as an intense burning, itching, sensation which comes and goes although sometimes the feeling is so overwhelming and intense that it is difficult to keep going on with your normal every day routine.

There is often redness and irritation of the labia (the genital "lips").

Pain during sexual intercourse.

A specific "yeasty" smell - this will be instantly recognizable as it will have the odor of beer or bread although the yeast in these foodstuffs is completely different to what we have in our bodies.

- Burning or pain during urination.

- A thick, white discharge from the vagina - this is unpleasant and can have the appearance and consistency of ricotta cheese although this is not necessarily true in all cases as it can be any consistency and can even be yellowish or clear.

The various symptoms of Candida are due to the toxins which are being released into the system. There are other physical indicators which can potentially but not always be present, some of these include:

- Cold hands / feet

- Low body temperature.

- Bad breath (halitosis)

- Coating on tongue (oral thrush)

- Constipation

- Diarrhea

- Dry mouth

- Intestinal system upsets.

- Acne

- Blurred vision

- Burning or tingling

- Chemical sensitivity

- Headaches

- Hives

- Muscle aches, pain, weakness and tension

- Nasal congestion

- Head tension

- Depression

- Fatigue

- Irritability

- Skin problems and random itches

- Urinary infections / problems

- Painful intercourse

The Importance of Getting a Doctors Diagnosis

It is of the utmost importance in the first instance to see a health professional to gain a preliminary diagnosis if you believe that you have a vaginal or oral yeast infection. It is important to identify what exactly you are dealing with so that you can make an informed decision with regards to the best road to go down with regards to treatment.

Always consult your doctor if you believe that you have a yeast infections and:

- You have never had one before

- You are suffering from recurrent infections

- Have never received a positive yeast infection diagnosis

There are studies which suggest that many women who purchase over the counter remedies and treatments for yeast infections actually do not even have one. In fact over use or using these medicines can lead to difficult to treat infections. This is why it is so important to be properly and expertly diagnosed. There are many STI's which mimic the symptoms of vaginal candidiasis and if these are left untreated then they can have a knock on effect on your general and sexual health. Some STI's have been known to cause infertility, problems in pregnancy and even to increase your risk of contracting gynecological cancers.

There are a few other conditions which present with symptoms similar to those of vaginal candidiasis:

- If you are suffering from a vaginal bacterial infection then this can present in a similar way to a yeast infection especially there is an itch or pain present. However, a big difference is that the vaginal discharge can present in some alarming looking colors such as dark yellow, green, or brown. Also the smell will be extremely unpleasant and tends to smell like rotting fish. Go to the doctor if you think that you may have a bacterial infection.

- Trichomoniasis is sexually transmitted and presents as an itch down below accompanied by pain on urination and abdominal pain. Intercourse may be uncomfortable also. This infection is caused by a parasite which can infect the vagina and also the urinary tract. See a medical professional if you think you may have the infection.

- A UTI (urinary tract infection) is caused by bacteria infecting the urethra and not the vagina. UTIs present with many symptoms such as chills, an ache or a feeling of pressure within the lower abdomen and / or back, burning and pain when urinating, a constant urge to urinate and mucus or blood in the urine. UTI's need to be caught early as if left untreated the infection can cause damage to the kidneys.

How Can I Minimize My Risk of Contracting a Yeast Infection?

There are many general rules with regards to minimizing your risk of contracting a yeast infection. To begin with, taking a look at something as simple as the clothes that you wear can help you avoid lots of potential problems. Yeast loves a warm and moist environment, in fact these are the optimum conditions in which is grows. Give nylon underwear and pantyhose without cotton gussets a miss. Avoid synthetic fabrics close to your private parts and don't wear those favorite skinny jeans every day! If you enjoy going to the gym then change into your tight lycra gear when you get there, wear cotton underwear and then get showered and changed into more loose fitting clothes as soon as you finish your class or workout. If you are a keen swimmer or are planning on doing a lot of swimming on holiday then don't lounge around in a wet swim suit!

Ensure that you shower often and that you dry the vaginal area thoroughly. As previously stated, wear cotton underwear whenever possible and in bed try not to wear any at all.

If you are unwell, whenever possible and obviously under the direction of your doctor, try not to take too many courses of antibiotics unless they are necessary. Also the birth control pill and steroids are best avoided if at all possible.

There are many natural herbal and nutritional supplements which women feel help keep yeast infections at bay. Encouraging good bacterial flora can be helped along with the help of a naturopath and by following a diet low in sugar, milk, fruit juices, refined sugars and also carbohydrates such as potatoes. Foods with a high yeast / mold content including cheese, alcoholic beverages, and dried fruits should also be avoided. You can work out what is best for you through trial and error. Too much sugar and carbohydrates which are converted to sugar in the body will only encourage the growth and development of a yeast infection.

If you are diabetic or suspect that you might be, ensure that your diabetes is well controlled and that your diet is balanced. The balanced diet rule applies to non diabetics too!

Another important rule for girls and women who are susceptible to yeast infections is that they should not use perfumed or colored soaps, lotions, bath gels etc and must avoid taking too many bubble baths. Douching is also a no no. Also you have to be careful with regards to what you use to wash your laundry and which sanitary protection you use. The rule with regards to products containing perfume is to do your best to avoid these and therefore avoid the risk of irritation.

Also, although Candida is not classed as a sexually transmitted disease you need to ensure than when having intercourse with your partner that you are both clean. If your partner is someone who is a little lazy with regards to hygiene and he is uncircumcised then you need to remember that he could have all sorts of little nasties hiding under there. Especially if he is an active person who is always on the go and doesn't have time to get showered and cleaned up as much as you would like. If he has a yeast problem and you are tired or run down and your immune system is low then you can potentially run the real risk of catching the infection from him. Remember also that you cannot necessarily see if he has an infection as he could have no symptoms at all. If you are in doubt about his hygiene level then why not buy him some nice toiletries or suggest that you both take a shower together. Or, if the subtle message just isn't getting through to him then you will just need to come out with it and tell him that it is just not on and that you need him to follow good hygiene rules for the benefit of you both. I know that this sounds harsh but you are potentially saving yourself from a great deal of upset, discomfort and potentially a long term infection too. Good luck!

Chapter 2: The Negative Impact It Has On Your Life

How a Yeast Infection Affects Your Day to Day Life

It is an unpleasant experience altogether to be suffering from a yeast infection. You may feel that everyone knows or that somehow they can tell. This is natural so don't panic or over worry about this. There is help and support online where you can find other women to either speak to or to read about who have had or are going through the exact same journey which you are on. This is one of the wonders of the modern age. Our mothers had to go through the experience of having a yeast infection entirely alone - that is unless they had close friends or relatives whom they could discuss things with. Luckily for us, there is so much information online and the stigma of conditions such as this is beginning to dissipate. So, if you are feeling lonely, upset or down then be assured that there are others out there feeling exactly the same and yet more women who lead full and fun lives in spite of their condition.

Even if normally you are a confident person then being diagnosed with any medical condition can have a detrimental effect on your confidence. Due to the nature of a yeast infection your usual happy attitude can take a blow and you must work harder to remain positive each and every day. You CAN beat this and you WILL! There are many ways of treating and managing this even when your condition is chronic or recurring. You just need to take your time and to find out what works best for you.

If you are experiencing real problems with regards to your confidence and self esteem or you are just generally feeling down then you should ask for help. Whether this is just from speaking with friends to get your feelings out or if in the case of depression, you need a little more help. See your doctor if you are having difficulty in living your day to day life due to feeling depressed. Signs to look out for include tiredness and irritability, loss of interest in life, sexual disinterest and a feeling of hopelessness. However feeling this way is rare and most people who have Candida get through it and resume feeling good about themselves.

When you have a yeast infection it is an idea to take changes of cotton underwear with you on days during which you are feeling very uncomfortable and itchy. Changing your panties regularly will make you feel and smell fresher if odor is a problem. Try buying some new and pretty cotton underwear which will make you feel good and be careful to thoroughly wash these regularly on a high temperature setting.

In rare cases, Candida overgrowth can lead to hair loss. The root cause of this affliction is not yet entirely clear but medical professionals have a few theories. The first is enzyme deficiency and enzyme suppression which is caused directly by Candida and can cause hair loss. Also a deficiency in essential fatty acids can lead to hair thinning, hair loss and dry and brittle hair. A yeast overgrowth can also cause thyroid dysfunction which in turn leads to the loss of ones hair. A lack of vitamins and minerals due to the fungal infection stopping the body from absorbing them can also cause the loss of hair and finally deep scarring of the skin due to the fungus can stop the hair growing as well as it should.

Don't worry about this though as Candida hair loss can be stopped with the correct treatment. Take vitamins and good probiotic supplements to replenish the good bacteria within your gut in order to absorb the right minerals which are required for healthy hair growth. It can be a long road and can take around between three and six months for your hair to begin to grow again and for most people there is a full recovery.

There is no reason why you can't live your life in the way in which you generally like to live it. Just ensure that you are prepared for eventualities and that you bring with you any treatment which you are currently using if you are out and about or at work. It is of paramount importance that you treat yourself regularly and continue to follow impeccable hygiene practices in order to eradicate the yeast overgrowth and to return your body to its usual happy self.

What About My Usual Routine?

A great way to lift yourself up when you are down with regards to this condition is to go out and spoil yourself. Try that new hair style, buy that new fashionable dress. Do whatever it takes for you to feel good and to feel happy about yourself. Also ensuring that all of this cotton underwear which you do buy is pretty and stylish will make you feel great. So consign those old grey, baggy panties to the bin and get with it! Meet up with friends, continue with your life. Having a yeast infection may force you to look at your lifestyle and how you can change this to perhaps make it healthier but it shouldn't stop your life.

When you do meet up with friends, don't be afraid to confide in them and to tell them how you are feeling. As women you all go through similar experiences and can support one another. When you do meet your friends, why not go out for lunch and eat a lovely healthy meal which will encourage the conditions within your body to eradicate that excess yeast. Avoid sugary and glutinous foods, and eat lots of protein rich dishes, lots of vegetables, live yogurt and seeds and oils. Don't go wild on the alcohol as this will only feed the yeast. Starchy foods are also a no no as this will only convert to sugar and will leave you back where you started. The great thing which will happen as a result of your diet change will be that you will be training your body up for the future. To avoid recurrences of Candida then it is a good idea to consistently follow a healthy diet.

Also ensure that you wash your used underwear regularly and at a higher temperature than usual. Ironing your underwear on a high heat is known to be a good way of ensuring that they remain sterile and cannot reinfect you. There are even stories about women who have sterilized their underwear in the microwave although this could pose a fire risk and therefore should be avoided!

Tight clothing needs to be avoided at all costs as it will only prolong and exacerbate the condition, loose trousers and flowing skirts can really help with the healing process.

If you are in a little pain with the condition then take some pain relief to relieve the discomfort if need be. Also remember that with this condition, early and regular treatment is very important. If you do leave the infection to go wild on its own then you will find that your symptoms can worsen and other problems can potentially ensue. Particularly with regards to pain and itching, so this is something to keep in mind.

Be careful with regards to getting too close to people you don't know the sexual history of also, this is a rule which applies to everyone - thrush is not exclusively passed on this way but you could contract it from a male or female who is already infected. Potentially you could contract something much more difficult to treat also and remember that both you and your partner if you have one will need treatment and a little abstinence from intercourse for a number of days.

Recurring Chronic Yeast Infection and You

Any woman who has ever had a yeast infection knows just how horrible they can be. You need to put up with pain, swelling, redness, itching, a constant discharge and a plethora of other symptoms. A chronic yeast infection means that you will have to contend with this over and over again and you may feel that you are at the end of your tether. There is only so much that one person can take and you may find that you need a complete lifestyle change and a whole rebalance of your body from the inside out in order to feel as you should again.

As we spoke about previously, physical illness can adversely affect your emotional and mental health. You may find that you are just tired out having to endure these uncomfortable symptoms regularly.

If you leave your Candida infection without treating it, suffer from chronic infection or are too embarrassed to seek help then you run the risk of more complications, more itchiness and swelling and also even open sores and cuts.

It is important to find out how your body responds to different treatments, many of which we will cover later. It is also important to remember that once you find out by a process of elimination what has been causing your condition, then you can work to balance this and to bring back good health to your body and mind.

Many women swear by colon cleansing or colonic irrigation to rid their bodies of all of the toxins and build ups which can encourage an overgrowth of yeast within your body.

An overgrowth of Candida can be helped considerably by being in a hot, dry climate as the sun destroys the fungus. Perhaps the best excuse possible for that holiday which you have your eye on! A holiday or a trip away can be very beneficial with regards to treating your emotional and mental state if you are suffering from a chronic infection as illness and imbalance drag you down. Due to the fact that you can become exhausted and mentally "foggy" with Candida then you need to look after your mental health particularly well. Also if you have a partner then it will give you time away together to get closer as you may not have been able to be physically close for some time due to your condition.

You CAN treat chronic Candida successfully.

How to Tell Your Partner?

It is very hard to talk about such "icky" and important issues with a partner. You may feel a sense of shame and embarrassment - don't worry as this is entirely natural and to be expected! Many many women have been in your shoes and they haven't died of embarrassment.

Men can get this infection too and although it is quite rare, it is actually possible for thrush to be passed through sexual intercourse. If he has a weakened immune system, or practices very poor personal bodily hygiene then a man is more likely to get the infection. Also uncircumcised men are more likely to get thrush due to the warmth and the damp environment under the foreskin. Potentially a couple can pass this back and forth over and over again so it is very important that you both get treated if you are in a relationship. You have a duty to tell a partner whether you are still together or not if you feel that you have had Candida whilst being sexually active with them.

What your fellow needs to watch out for is inflammation of the head of the penis and also general inflammation in the foreskin area. Also your partner will be putting up with a very uncomfortable and tender sensation on his private parts. He will likely also feel very itchy too and may have a discharge from the tip of his penis. Also be aware that you could have been infected by him in the first place although it is more likely that you have an imbalance within your body. If your partner presents with any of these symptoms then he will need to be treated as soon as possible.

A yeast infection is called Candida Balanitis in men and it can potentially remain undiagnosed for years. Unlike its female version which presents with many unpleasant symptoms, a male yeast infection can quite often be asymptomatic, that is it will not show any actual symptoms. Alternatively it can manifest through general and non specific blotches which are inconclusive. Statistics tell that on average men are less likely than women to develop the infection.

So, how to tell your partner? If you are close enough to be having sex together then you should be able to talk to one another about anything. If you feel that you cannot approach him then you need to think of alternative means. Bring up the subject with him casually, say that a friend has had it in the past and explain that this is just a natural imbalance within the body. Explain also that it is not a sexually transmitted disease but that he will probably need treatment too so that you don't pass the infection between you. There is a risk through oral and genital sex so it is very important that you both get this taken care of as soon as you can.

If you and your partner are close and talk a lot and in depth about everything in life then telling him will be easier. Just approach this in conversation and tell him, explain the facts and allay his fears as you will be beginning to become very well informed about the condition now. It might be a good idea for you both to read something like this together to answer any questions which he may have because whilst Candida is an every day word for women, it doesn't affect men as much and he may have heard all manner of wrong information about the condition.

Now that you have told him, give it time to settle in to his mind.

The Big Question - Is It Safe To Have Sex Whilst Infected?

Studies show that rarely men can contract a yeast infection from their female partner. However studies also show that practicing good hygiene after sex negates the possibility of the yeast infection transferring. It needs to be noted that some women who have very severe yeast infections can find it rather painful to have sex whilst infected. Some find that it helps to shower thoroughly beforehand and to use some anti thrush preparation during intercourse. It is normal for the vagina to burn a little during sex if you have this infection and you may feel more comfortable if you refrain from intercourse.

If both parties are happy with going ahead then you can theoretically go ahead and have sex so long as the man washes his full genital area very thoroughly afterwards. Males can carry yeast on and around their private parts for several days and there is the potential for this to be passed back to the woman. Most couples prefer not to have sex and many doctors would agree with this. It is better to wait until the infection is completely cured just to be as safe as possible, especially if you suffer from painful chronic or recurring thrush.

If a male gives oral sex to his partner who has a yeast infection then it is not 100% likely to transfer to the male but if his system is low with regards to immunity, for example, if he has HIV, cancer etc, then he can potentially contract it. It is therefore safer and perhaps more pleasant for both parties to refrain from oral activities until the infection has fully cleared up.

Interestingly, receiving oral sex has been linked to an increase with regards to women getting yeast infections. The best thing to do is to seek advice from your doctor and if he advises you to hold off on any practices then do as he says. You want to get rid of the infection as quickly as possible.

Potentially at any one time there is a very high percentage of Americans who are carrying a yeast infection at any one time and a significant number of these individuals don't even realize it.

With regards to your partner, if he is infected he may not even know it as more often than not Candida in a male does not show any symptoms or the symptoms are so vague that he really doesn't pay much attention! The condition can manifest itself as rashes, blisters, itchy bumps, blisters and dry cracks which will show on the tip of the penis. He may be aware of an intense and burning sensation on urination. Sometimes these symptoms can become so bad and so annoying and uncomfortable that they can wake the sufferer during the night. There can also be a thick white discharge present although this is not always so. If you or your partner are worried about that likelihood that he may have a fungal infection then the best thing to do is to get him checked out by the doctor. You want to rule out anything else and to get him set on the best course of treatment for him. The problem which you now face though is getting him to see the doctor in the first instance and then to show the doctor the problem! Men are notoriously shy of visiting the doctor and are nowhere near as used to having their private areas examined as ladies are!

You know what it is like - due to decades upon decades of social conditioning men like to prove that they are tough guys and are even taught from a very young age that they have to be tough and that complaining about their health or showing any non butch signs is a weakness. Now us ladies know that this is all nonsense but it is difficult to reprogram your man - you will no doubt be nodding your head in agreement as you read this! What your man needs to know however is that this "old school" way of thinking has been perpetualizing and exacerbating mens health problems probably since the dawning of human life on earth. So many hours of pain, suffering and worrying could have been saved if only our men had been prepared to visit the doctor although todays man is far better at this that his father and grandfather ever were. Because of fear, social conditioning, ignorance and even denial of their conditions men have worried about going to visit the doctor. A great way to get your husband used to this, if he is not a modern and health conscious fellow, is to bring him along to the doctor with you, let him wait in the waiting room for you and let him see that there is nothing at all to worry about. He will soon realize how silly he has been and will take better care of his health.

Remember whilst taking the decision whether or not to have intercourse whilst infected that it can take between a few weeks and as long as a month or more to be clear of the yeast infection. If you are potentially and continuously infecting one another back and forth then this will take far longer to clear and can even cause more problems. Think about what is best for you both as a couple and remember that the infection will go and that you can resume normal life soon.

Chapter 3: Modern Medicine Isn't Always Best

A Doctor's Diagnosis and Conventional Testing

There are regular doctor's tests which will diagnose whether or not you have the Candida infection present within your body. The facts are that some females who have thrush do not exhibit many or even any signs and symptoms. In these cases the infection may only be picked up by chance when attending for a pap test.

In the first instance you are always best to get a conventional doctor's diagnosis and in the future you will be aware of the signs to look out for in the case that your body is out of balance again and a yeast overgrowth ensues.

Sometimes your doctor will just interview you and ask you about your symptoms in order to determine whether you have Candida. Thrush is not categorized as sexually transmitted, so your partner will not need to be tested unless they exhibit symptoms.

Most often though if he wishes to rule out anything else or if you have recently had unprotected intercourse he offer you a test.

There are various ways in which you can be clinically tested for a yeast infection:

- **A Simple Swab Test**

This is a simple procedure which is pain free and involves a sample of the cells in your vagina being taken with a cotton swab which is then sent to a laboratory for analysis. The good aspect of taking this test is that it will show also if your symptoms are being caused by other conditions, for example trichomonas or bacterial vaginosis.

- **Blood Test**

This is a test which checks for the three antibodies which show your immune system's reaction to Candida. The antibodies are called IgG, IgA, and IgM. If there are high levels of these within the blood then this is an indication that there is an overgrowth of Candida.

- **Stool Analysis**

This is just as it sounds and a sample of your stool will be checked for yeast, friendly bacteria and also unfriendly pathogenic bacteria. You can also submit this test by post to a lab and this will be a good way to indicate if there is an overgrowth of yeast within your body. It can also detect conditions such as parasitic infections which can present in a similar way and with similar symptoms.

- **Urine Tartaric Acid Test**

This is a very useful test which detects tartaric acid within your urine. Tartaric acid is a waste product of Candida overgrowth therefore if you have a high level of this within your sample then you have a yeast overgrowth present within your body.

With any of these medical Candida tests, you will need to visit the doctor and then they will order the tests. The next step after testing is for the specimens to be sent to a laboratory and then the results will be forwarded on to your doctor. A second visit with the doctor will then be scheduled in order for you to be given your results. At this appointment the doctor will discuss treatment options with you.

Self Diagnosis

There are many women, especially ones who know their bodies and who are prone to having yeast infections who understand their symptoms and recognize that they are suffering from an attack. In this instance it is common for a woman to self diagnose although a first diagnosis with the doctor is generally recommended. There are a few ways in which to test yourself for the presence of an overgrowth of yeast. Here are the two most common:

Spit Test

The Spit Test is a very simple test which you can do quickly in the home, without having to go out and buy any specialist equipment and without having to spend money.

- On waking in the morning, even before you go to brush your teeth and before you eat or drink, fill a glass with room temperature bottled water.

- Spit a little of your saliva into the glass.

- Check the contents of the glass every twenty minutes or so for approximately an hour.

If you see any of these signs then it is likely that you have a Candida infection:

- If there are strings of saliva reaching down through the water from the saliva which is still at the top

- If your saliva is looking cloudy and is settled on the bottom of the glass

- If you detect opaque looking little specks of saliva which are suspended in the water

If you have never had Candida before or you are worried that you could have picked up something from someone then do go to your doctor for a proper diagnosis.

Online

There are online sites offering testing at a price and with these you usually send off your money, test yourself using a kit which the lab send out to you and then mail them a sample back.

There are also in depth questionnaires online which will assess your symptoms to tell if you have the likelihood of having a Candida overgrowth. Obviously this type of self diagnosis is inconclusive and if you are worried or in doubt then you should seek medical advice.

Signs and Symptoms

Of course a great way in which to tell if you have Candida is to see if you have the symptoms of this. Do remember however that other disorders and infections can present with symptoms which are very similar to those of Candida so if you are in doubt or have never had an "official" diagnosis then you do need to go and see a doctor.

Here are some of the symptoms of Candida overgrowth:

- Frequent stomach pains
- Digestion problems
- Skin problems
- Difficulty concentrating
- Constant tiredness
- Exhaustion
- Anxiety
- Headaches
- Obsessive compulsive disorder
- Anger outbursts
- Irritability
- Mood swings
- Intense cravings for sugars and yeasty products

- Itchy skin

Modern Medicine to Treat Thrush

Modern medicine has given us so many wonderful advances but when it comes to treating Candida then less is definitely more. You have to be careful that you don't take too many courses of antibiotics and creams as your yeast infection, if it recurs can become resistant to treatment. Also antibiotics have a known yeast encouraging effect within your body.

Conventional treatments can kill off some of the friendly bacteria within your system so if you go down this route then look to the alternative health community to help balance your system. Taking a probiotic will help, but more about that later.

If you have particularly mild symptoms then your doctor will generally recommend a short antifungal medicine course which will last for approximately one to three days. However if your symptoms are chronic or severe then your course of treatment will be lengthier.

There are a variety of conventional treatment options which are available through the doctor and also to buy over the counter. These include taking tablets orally, using a cream or inserting pessaries into your vagina. There is no real difference between the effects of taking tablets or pessaries.

Your either buy these treatments over the counter or you can be prescribed them by your doctor.

Tablets

In its tablet form fluconazole is usually used as an antifungal treatment. This treatment is often extremely effective with just one tablet often being enough to completely cure an attack. The downside of this treatment is that it can potentially cause side-effects such as nausea and vomiting, constipation, bloating and / or diarrhea. Special care must be taken if you are pregnant or breastfeeding or even think that you could perhaps be pregnant as there is a chance that these treatments could have an effect on your baby.

Pessaries

These generally do not cause the amount of side-effects that tablets do. On the down side they can be messy to use, can potentially cause damage to diaphragms and condoms and can cause local irritation. Again there are pregnancy warnings which come with the use of these. Pregnant women should not use the applicator to insert pessaries in case of injury to the cervix. Instead they must insert the pessary by hand.

Creams

Creams can be used along with the two aforementioned forms of treatment to treat any redness and soreness in the vaginal and vulval areas.

Conventional Vs. Holistic Treatment

More and more women are turning to natural cures and treatments for Candida. They may have tried prescription or over the counter conventional medications and these treatment options may simply not have proved helpful. In some cases perhaps the drugs provided short term relief only for the the symptoms of the infection to return (chronic thrush).

There is a high percentage of women who have used conventional cures for yeast infections only for the symptoms to come back with a vengeance after a temporary lull or even an absence. In some documented cases their infection has come back and become even worse.

Nowadays and with so much information being available on the internet, people are becoming increasingly aware of any potentially negative or harmful effects of using conventional treatments. Many individuals worry that these drugs may have a detrimental effect on the smooth functioning of the bodies immune and natural defense systems.

The action of the long term use of pharmaceutical medications which prove to be ineffective, can actually lower the natural immunity of the body, making it more open to yeast infections. Obviously this is a completely opposite effect to what one wishes to happen and there are many anecdotal reports of sufferers of yeast infection who have spent considerable amounts of their money and also their time on drug treatments only to have little or no joy.

The holistic community believe that it is best to begin with understanding the catalyst which makes these infections begin within the body and to address these rather than solely treating the end result as conventional treatments do. The holistic view makes sense with regards to any ailment or physical problem. Until the underlying cause is addressed and treated correctly the symptoms will not get any better and could potentially worsen.

When a holistic approach to an illness or infection is embarked upon, you will be changing and looking at all aspects of your lifestyle such as diet, exercise and emotional health - everything. You will be taking a look at the bigger picture and changing your life and stress levels in order to bring balance and health into your life for the longterm. A holistic approach works on the root cause of an imbalance and on how to rid yourself of the yeast infection forever whereas conventional treatments work at eradicating only the symptoms whenever they arise.

Reported Side Effects of Conventional Treatments.

Unfortunately, many of the conventional treatmebts for Candida may cause patients to suffer from side effects such as diarrhea, abdominal pain, nausea, hives, swelling, itching, rashes and potentially a drop in blood pressure. These side effects if they present only add to the feelings of ill health which are already afflicting the Candida sufferer.

Another important consideration is the fact that many drugs can react with one another and create dangerous side effects. You must always tell your doctor if you are taking any other medications if you begin a new course of anti yeast treatment so that he can ascertain as to whether there are any potential contraindications.

As well as the potentially hazardous side effects from using prescription drugs for Candida, many of the treatments can even exacerbate the condition as some of them contain sugar which encourages yeast proliferation and can also render the treatment unsuitable for diabetics.

Anti-thrush tablets which are prescribed by doctors for vaginal Candida contain antifungal medicines. Anti-thrush tablets can potentially cause side effects, including:

- an upset stomach
- vomiting
- headache
- diarrhea
- constipation
- wind
- bloating
- nausea

Vaginal pessaries exhibit less potential side effects then the tablets, but they can:

- be difficult to use and to get the hang of
- leave stains on your underwear (they do wash out)
- cause redness, a mild burning sensation and itching
- damage diaphragms and latex condoms (another form of contraception should be used whilst under this treatment)

- You shouldn't overuse vaginal pessaries as if you keep getting infections over and over there could be an underlying cause, for example other medicines or diabetes or potentially you have an infection which is not actually Candida.

What to do if you're pregnant or breastfeeding:

If you are pregnant or breastfeeding and have Candida or suspect that you may have it then you must always visit your doctor for help and advice rather than buying over the counter medication. You will be unable to take oral tablets due to their potential effects on your baby and you will likely be given a pessary which means that you will need to take care when inserting it so that you do not injure your cervix. To reduce this risk, always insert the pessaries manually as opposed to using the applicator provided. A cream may be prescribed if you have external symptoms such as itching and redness.

Chapter 4: Getting Rid of It Without pharmaceuticals

What is a Holistic Approach?

The definition of the word "holistic" is "relating to or concerned with wholes or complete systems rather than with the analysis of, treatment of, or dissection into parts -- medicine which attempts to treat both the mind and the body."

For a true holistic approach, we must consider the WHOLE being, including the emotional, mental, and physical. Holistic approaches include Herbalism, Acupuncture, Ayurveda, Homeopathy and Traditional Chinese Medicine.

Whereas the conventional medical establishment generally views the body as a collection of isolated parts rather than as a whole, holistically speaking it is very different. Conventional treatments are often aimed at suppressing and not eliminating symptoms. Holistic speaking we are taught to listen to our bodies as symptoms which it exhibits are regarded as the body expressing imbalance and a need to return to homeostasis (a state of equilibrium). The suppression of symptoms is believed to manifest as new and potentially more serious problems and conditions in other areas. Holistic treatments center around assisting the body to heal itself by finding out and then eliminating the underlying cause(s) of the problem. These can be either physical, environmental, behavioral etc. or a combination of these.

It is important to note that even holistic practitioners urge individuals not shun all conventional medicine as there are many situations where it is a necessity to be treated by a qualified medical doctor.

It is important to be aware of the possibility of holistic therapies having the ability to be just as capable of suppression of symptoms as conventional medicines so if you are looking to introduce any of these methods and practices into your life in order to eradicate your Candida then you need to take advice.

It is important to research any big change within your life, especially when it will have an effect upon your health and well being. Holistic health is all about multi-dimensional healing, as opposed to specific medicines for specific cures. It looks after the well being of and takes into account the affect illness and stress has on the body, mind, emotions, & spirit.

A Holistic Cure For Candida?

Many women who wish to treat their bodies without harsh modern medicines are looking for a holistic cure for thrush. Perhaps the conventional yeast infection medications have not worked for them as is the case for many chronic thrush sufferers. The great news is that there exist a range of holistic treatments and potential cures which can help restore the inner balance of your body.

Vaginal yeast infections can be treated by getting to the root of what is causing them. This includes modifying the way you eat and your way of life.

One of the biggest and most important changes you will have to make is in your diet. This may be extremely difficult for many women as our eating habits have been with us for the whole of our lives but if you work hard at making real changes then you will find that it has been worth the hassle. Yeast overgrows within the body for many reasons, mainly though this is due to an improper diet or a stressful lifestyle. The main change which you are going to have to make is to eradicate sugar from your diet, at least for a while, usually for approximately three months. Doing this will help to kill the yeast fungus within your body as you will not be feeding it. Another big change which you will need to make is to avoid processed foods as much as possible and to replace them with a diet which is rich in fresh vegetables and fruits. This will help to flush the toxins the yeast fungus out of your system.

It is also important to avoid external factors which can exacerbate the condition such as stress, too many antibiotics, certain chemicals and birth control. Probiotics such as live unsweetened yogurt or acidophilus will help. Taking these in conjunction with herbal remedies and topical herbal tinctures and creams can in many cases clear the problem. Probiotics are incredibly useful and effective for both healing and also avoiding Candida overgrowth. Probiotics help nourish the 'good' flora in your intestines. Foods with probiotic actions include sauerkraut and fermented seed cheeses. Taken every day, probiotics will help keep your intestinal flora in balance.

Many women turn to treatments such as Homeopathy for help. Homeopathy is the name for a system of medicine which centers on treating a patient with extremely diluted substances. These on the whole are given mainly in tablet form and the aim if the treatment is to trigger the body's own natural systems of healing. A homeopath will match the most appropriate medicine to each patient dependant on their symptoms.

The whole principle of this method of healing is that you can treat 'like with like'. What this basically means is that a substance which causes adverse symptoms when taken in large doses, can therefore be used in minute, trace amounts to then treat those same symptoms. This thinking is at times used in conventional medicine. Sometimes small doses of allergens such as pollen are sometimes used in order to de-sensitize patients who suffer from allergies.

Homeopaths have several different ways and treatments for controlling chronic yeast infections, and they will tailor each type of regimen depending on the symptoms present and also depending on the individual. Often a homeopath will recommend belladonna and chamomilla for inflammation, borax to sooth the mucous membranes, and kreosotum or arsenicum album for itching and burning sensations.

It is especially beneficial for people who have chronic and recurring Candidal infections to follow the whole body holistic approach. Many women swear by colon cleansing or colonic irrigation to rid their bodies of all of the toxins and build ups which can encourage an overgrowth of yeast within your body. A chronic sufferer will get many bouts of yeast infection throughout the year and generally over the counter and prescription medicine will not work for them as the infection will just keep recurring. Often women who are in this predicament are so desperate that they will try anything to shift it. Through following a few simple lifestyle changes then you can change your life and you can be free of this millstone around your neck. You can beat Candida if you treat the root cause and not solely the symptoms.

The Importance of a Good Diet

Without exception, the most important aspect of the holistic approach is a healthy diet. No treatments, whether holistic or conventional, will truly be of complete benefit if you do not intake the necessary nourishment for the body to do its work.

An anti Candida diet is one which is very simply put together. To begin with one must ensure that in the first instance you cleanse and flush out your system in order to eradicate toxins. Thereafter you must begin a strict diet free from foods such as the ones on this list: mature / aged cheeses, alcohol, dried fruits, chocolate, fresh fruits, mushrooms, fermented foods, vinegar, wheat, rye, barley, sugar, honeys and syrups and foods that contain yeast or mold such as breads, muffins and cakes. When you begin this diet you must begin taking probiotics and antifungals also. Once the Candida overgrowth has been eradicated then you will be able to reintroduce foods slowly, watching for any detrimental health effects as you go.

Good foods to eat are vegetables (including a great amount of raw garlic which is a strong anti fungal agent), protein (beef, chicken, eggs, fish), live yogurt cultures (both dairy and non dairy), acidophilus, green algae such as spirulina and chlorella, nuts, seeds and oils, and non-glutinous grains such as millet, rice, rice bran and oat bran.

Aloe Vera juice/gel and also coconut oil are both very beneficial for the intestinal flora. They are soothing and balancing. Also drinking green vegetable juices will encourage your system to be in balance.

The use within the diet of anti-fungal agents like grapefruit seed extract, pau d'arco, fresh garlic, oil of oregano and tea tree oil will help combat Candida directly as opposed to being a preventative and soothing measure.

To complement the dietary changes which you are making, ensure that you are getting enough vitamins A, B complex and C, zinc, iron and magnesium within your diet.

- Direct measures which will help combat Candida are eating up to eight ounces of plain live yogurt every day. Also inserting a tampon which is coated in plain live yogurt within your vagina and leaving for half an hour or so will soothe your symptoms as the beneficial bacteria will have time to be absorbed into the body.

- To relieve Candida symptoms you can drink a mix of one teaspoon of apple cider vinegar, a quarter of a cup of warm water and a teaspoon of honey with each meal.

- Caprylic acid is a fatty acid with antibacterial qualities and which is naturally occurring. Take the standard dose daily with meals.

- Garlic supplements are great to combat Candida especially if you cannot stomach raw garlic.

Spirulina

Spirulina is a blue green algae which grows naturally under extreme conditions such as within volcanic lakes. Also it is grown commercially for use in tablets and powders.

Spirulina is a "miracle" supplement for increasing health and vitality. Also, it works great if you are looking to eliminate Candida as it contains so many nutrients and vitamins which will support your system.

Studies have indicated the strong anti-viral properties which the supplement has. In trials it has protected mice from strains of the HIV virus. Spirulina works by strengthening the immune system along with its enzymes which repair DNA which could prevent certain cancers from forming.

Spirulina as a regularly taken supplement has been proven to promote the growth of good intestinal bacterial flora which inhibits Candida from overgrowing. Spirulina also strengthens the immune system thus discouraging Candida cells to overgrow.

It is important to note however that you need to ensure that you buy only high quality Spirulina supplements. Look for the name "Arthrospira platensis".

Three grams of Spirulina contains:

- Protein 2 g
- Vitamin A (Beta Carotene)
- Vitamin B-1 (Thiamin)
- Vitamin B-2 (Riboflavin)
- Niacin B vitamin
- Folate (as folic acid)
- Vitamin B-12
- Iron
- Phosphorus
- Magnesium
- Phycocyanin
- Linolenic Acid
- Gamma Linolenic Acid
- Chlorophyll
- Carotenoids
- Superoxide Dismutase
- Omega-3 Fatty Acids include alpha linolenic acid
- Boron mineral.

Herbs and Supplements

The following supplements have been through clinical trials which have proven them to be effective with regards to treating thrush. The suggested usage period is a period of three months, after which the dosage or continuation can be looked at and assessed depending on your new condition.

Important note: You must not ingest any of the following herbs if you currently taking a course of HRT or any other hormonal treatment unless this is under the guidance of a registered practitioner.

Taking a good multivitamin and mineral supplement is the basis of any supplement program. This ensures that you are setting a firm foundation to ensure optimum health. To this you can add:

Zinc:

Women who are deficient in zinc seem to acquire recurrent thrush. Zinc is needed for a well functioning immune system and those who are deficient in zinc are known to be susceptible to recurrent infections.

Probiotics:

A probiotic is the complete opposite of an antibiotic therefore it encourages good bacteria rather than destroying bad bacteria within the body. Yoghurt is helpful in preventing attacks of yeast overgrowth, but probiotics can actually treat the yeast infection. This is because the lactobacillus levels within yoghurt are high enough to prevent thrush, but they are not enough to control an infection.

Beta-carotene:

There are low levels of beta-carotene in the vaginal cells of women who have thrush therefore a supplement may help to balance this.

Essential Fatty Acids:

These are found in nuts, seeds and oily fish and have wonderful anti-fungal, anti-bacterial and anti-viral properties and are therefore a very important weapon in your anti fungal attack.

Garlic:

Garlic is has been used as natures own antibiotic since ancient times and it is known for its positive effects on the immune system. It has antibacterial and anti-fungal properties and is good for prevention and also treatment of Candida. Clinical studies have shown that garlic extracts can prevent the growth of Candida. Allicin is one of the active ingredients within garlic and it is this which possesses the ability to prevent yeast overgrowth. It is therefore recommended that you buy supplements which contain high levels of this ingredient.

Herbs:

Herbal treatment is primarily aimed with the intention of treating an attack of thrush which is currently active and also on working to prevent further attacks.

Tea tree oil:

Research shows that tea tree oil is an excellent anti-fungal and antibacterial agent with regards to Candida. Try adding a few drops to your bath both as a treatment and also as a preventative measure. You can even buy tea tree oil pessaries which you can use as directed on the packaging.

Echinacea:

Echinacea is renowned for the positive effects that it has upon the immune system. Due to the fact that the immune system is compromised if you suffer with thrush and chronic thrush taking Echinacea is effective if taken with short breaks. For example, taking four weeks on and then one week off.

Chapter 5: Keeping It Away For Good

So now you know all about Candida. You have all the facts at your fingertips and you know how to eradicate this yeast overgrowth from your body. There is a lot of information within this book for you to take in so let's take a look at the main points:

- Think you have Candida? Then look out for these symptoms in particular -

Itching of the vulval and vaginal areas

A thick white discharge which can be likened to "cottage cheese"

Pain or burning upon urination and / or sexual intercourse

Extreme and unexplained tiredness

Bloating and gastrointestinal symptoms and upsets

A "spaced out" feeling

A dry mouth

Menstrual upsets

- Always ensure that you wear cotton underwear, loose clothing, that you don't use perfumes near the vaginal area, that you don't take too many courses of antibiotics or do anything else which may encourage an imbalance of yeast within the body

- If this is your first experience of what you believe is a yeast overgrowth then visit your doctor for a diagnosis. Also visit your doctor if there is a chance that you could have contracted the infection from another person via intercourse.

- If you have a partner, let them know your diagnosis so that they can see if they have any symptoms. They may need to be treated too.

- Look at the treatment options and decide on what you feel will be best for your wellbeing in both the long and the short term.

- Adjust your diet and cut out all sugars and carbohydrates which turn to sugar - this may take time and lots of willpower!

- Add probiotics and supplements to your diet. Garlic is especially effective against Candida

- It is natural to feel overwhelmed and even scared at times. This is not a journey which you have to go through alone and there are many support groups and online communities which can help.

- As time goes on you will feel your energy and zest for life returning. Congratulations, you are beating that yeast!

- Make your new lifestyle a permanent change as getting to the root of the problem will eradicate the yeast overgrowth forever.

- Don't panic, you CAN beat this and go back to living a normal, happy and fulfilling life!

Exclusive Bonus Download: Gluten Free Living Secrets

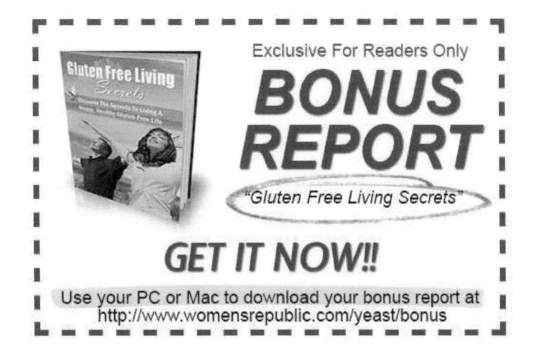

Download your bonus, please visit the download link above from your PC or MAC. To open PDF files, visit http://get.adobe.com/reader/ to download the reader if it's not already installed on your PC or Mac. To open ZIP files, you may need to download WinZip from http://www.winzip.com. This download is for PC or Mac ONLY and might not be downloadable to kindle.

Are you sick and tired of trying every weight loss program out there and failing to see results? Or are you frustrated with not feeling as energetic as you used to despite what you eat? Perhaps you always seem to have a bit of a " dodgy stomach " and indigestion seems to be a regular part of your life?

There's nothing worse than sitting down to a nice big plate of pasta and enjoying your meal only to be met with a growling stomach and the inevitable rush to the toilet.

It's that bloated feeling you get after eating a piece of bread that just " doesn't seem right " . Almost as if you've eaten something poisonous.

Gluten Free Living Secrets is a complete resource that will tell you everything you need to know about the dangers of eating gluten and how to go about transitioning yourself and your family to a life free of this dangerous substance.

Here's just a taste of what you will discover inside Gluten Free Living Secrets:

- What foods you should focus on when first switching to a gluten-free diet

- The 9 grains that are safe and gluten-free

- The truth about whether you can eat pasta on a gluten-free diet

- What you should know to determine if you have Celiac Disease

- and that's not all...

- Why you may want to consider eliminating gluten from your child's diet

- The top 10 reasons to go gluten-free

- How to transform your pantry to be gluten-free

- A list of essential gluten-free shopping tips

- How to keep your kids happy around their gluten-eating friends

- Tips on staying gluten-free when eating out

Gluten Free Living Secrets comes in a digital PDF format that is easy to read either on your computer or on your eBook reader.

Visit the URL above to download this guide and start achieving your overall health and weight loss goals NOW

One Last Thing...

Thank you so much for reading my book. I hope you really liked it. As you probably know, many people look at the reviews on Amazon before they decide to purchase a book. If you liked the book, could you please take a minute to leave a review with your feedback? 60 seconds is all I'm asking for, and it would mean the world to me.

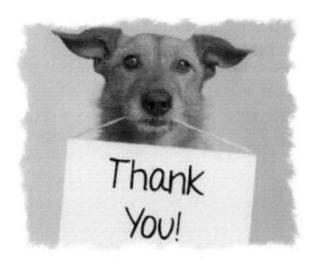

******

Books by This Author:

Permanently Beat Bacterial Vaginosis

Permanently Beat Yeast Infection & Candida

Permanently Beat Urinary Tract Infections

Permanently Beat Hypothyroidism Naturally

Permanently Beat PCOS

About the Author

Caroline D. Greene is a mother of 2 wonderful girls and a wife to a supportive husband. She has dedicated the past seven years to researching the various women's health topics that are not being openly discussed and providing help and support to the women dealing with these issues in their daily life.

Caroline D. Greene

Published by Women's Republic

Atlanta, Georgia USA

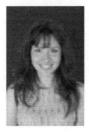

Printed in Great Britain
by Amazon.co.uk, Ltd.,
Marston Gate.